Education and Alternative Treatments for ADHD

Dr Giora Ram

IMEXCO General
Publishing
Israel

Education and Alternative Treatments for ADHD

Dr Giora Ram

First published in Israel by IMEXCO General Ltd.

Second edition

Printed in Israel

ISBN-13: 978-9659162369
ISBN-10: 9659162367

http://adhd.imexco.com

Table of Contents

1. PROLOGUE.

*What cannot be achieved with love
can be achieved with more love* (author).

THIS BOOK was written as a co-production of a special child and his father. It is based on extensive research on ADHD and its variations. The original book in Hebrew was entitled *ADHD - Children of Tomorrow*, published in Israel [2010].

Part of that book had naive stories in Hebrew and drawings made by the child, whilst the other part contained clinical analysis, practical suggestions and tools for parents in similar situations to enhance the important link between parents and their children. A unique methodological non-drug-based treatment successfully implemented on the author's son is presented here in conjunction with global education related issues.

The father-author carried out scientific activities for over the last three decades at the Weizmann Institute of Science at Rehovot, Israel, the Royal Postgraduate Medical School, London, the European Space Research Organization, Darmstadt, and the Keck Center for Collaborative Neuroscience at Rutgers University, New Jersey.

Dr Giora Ram

2. Drugs and the System.

Autism, ADD, ADHD, Asperger, Clonex, Dyslexia, Ritalin, Concerta, Adderall, Risperdal and are words that most readers will be familiar with, painfully familiar, if somebody in their family has been diagnosed with a specific syndrome or disorder and medically treated.

We will focus on those diagnoses and treatments not necessarily known to most of the population affected.

The clinical classification of our children into labelled categories could be seen as part of a conspiracy.

The education system, the medical system and the pharmaceutical companies form an unusual and aggressive cooperative in treating our labelled and classified children.

The three organizations share a symbiotic interest. The education system seeks *teachers' silence* so it will not need to cope with children with special needs.

The pharmaceutical companies have obvious monetary interests and use the medical profession to assist them in marketing and promoting their drugs.

Not surprisingly, most parents cooperate with them, as they think that if the paediatrician or the family doctor recommends certain treatment it must be for the benefit of their child.

It is important to emphasize that the author is not against medical treatment and in most cases medication is needed and justified.

The ambiguity and the broad spectrum of inaccurate diagnosis require investigation. This applies to most of the Western world, including, to a certain extent, the UK.

If we accept the current definitions of Attention Deficit Disorder (ADD) syndrome, then probably most of the population falls into this category.

This alone will increase false treatments, which may have unnecessary and sometimes harmful effects.

Moreover, it seems that this wide classification into groups requiring medication is also in the interests of the newly created profession of caretakers.

The proof is in the large number of psychotherapists, coaches and other so-called experts who have emerged in the last decade in a number of guises. To all that we can add the obvious interests of the pharmaceutical companies.

Obviously, there are cases genuinely requiring treatment and certain children will react positively, but there is concern about those who will be affected for life by wrong classifications and harmful medication.

3. Diagnosis and Treatment.

The need to diagnose both children and adults and classify them in the appropriate categories is diversified.

Legal, clinical and educational needs must be analysed and reported to the appropriate authorities. The increase in supply exceeds the increase in demand for the experts and institutions available and it seems that the entire population requires diagnosis.

It is essential to derive a diagnostic method which can minimize false positives, and especially to distinguish between sufferers of real syndromes and those who show certain signs of the said syndrome but are actually considered to be normal. Below are examples of cases which only experienced professionals can diagnose correctly.

- Evolutionary defects, seen in children with study difficulties such as attention deficit, may look similar to those evidenced in the ADD syndrome.

- Emotional situations that may cause attention problems, such as children under stress, abuse, neglect or other distress.
- Temperamental children maybe wrongly diagnosed as hyperactive although they are within the moderated hyperactivity range.
- Chronic disease, sleeping disorder, hearing or sight problems and malnourishment may cause misdiagnosis.
- Mental polarities such as genius or retardation may be interpreted as ADD.
- Behavioural disorder such as lack of motivation to study or insubordination may be interpreted as ADD.
- Fear or panic disorder that may be expressed as hyperactivity and attention difficulty like fear of failing in school.
- Depression disorder that is expressed in decline in activity, social disconnection and nervous and irritated moods is a case for misinterpretation.

The frenzied diagnosis and treatment applied by institutes and individual care providers is obvious from the many internet forums on the subject.

Worried parents visit numerous care providers, until they find the one who will supply them with the diagnosis that they seek. Given the large number of professionals available, they will certainly find one to support their diagnosis.

There is an endless and inappropriate war between school-appointed professionals and parents regarding the need to transfer children to the special education system. It exists everywhere where there are such options for the special education system but is particularly prevalent in the Western world.

The prejudice of such an education system, inflicting guilt and personal failure upon parents, means they try to resist the recommended change.

4. DRUGS AND CHILD'S BRAIN.

RITALIN, CONCERTA, ADDERALL, Risperdal and Clonex are only some of the drugs prescribed for our children by psychiatrists.

All this is in addition to vitamins, food supplements and over-the-counter drugs which are available without prescription and whose efficacy is questionable.

Ritalin, for example, is a stimulant which is very similar to cocaine. Long-term use can cause undesirable changes in a child's brain.

Dopamine is a neurotransmitter or a nerve conductive stimulant. It is a chemical substance in the brain that has a significant impact on attention and concentration. When concentrating, most children experience a substantial reduction in sugar and oxygen levels.

In those conditions of deficit, children look for excitement, which is sometimes dangerous, for the purpose of increasing their dopamine level.

The brain's need for extra dopamine makes children search for stimulating and exciting activities. The best and the healthiest way to increase dopamine levels naturally is by controlled physical activity. Obviously, there are medications to achieve that target as well, but these are not recommended as a first resort.

Over-exposure to dopamine may cause hallucinations and visual phenomena, which are typical symptoms of schizophrenia.

A very interesting phenomenon relates to the brain's need for dopamine.

There is a clear correlation between children with special needs and their skill in music and drawing. We can explain that phenomenon by the extra dopamine generated during those pleasurable activities.

Ritalin and cocaine affect the dopamine system which helps to control functioning of the brain during experiences of pleasure. The subject of side-effects is very problematic, especially for long-term drug treatments.

Here is a somewhat graphic description of what is going on in a child's brain when s/he is receiving certain medication.

The brain contains nerve cells or neurons. Each one of those neurons generates connections called synapses. The connections are enabled by electro-chemical communication.

We know that the more we learn, the more those connections increase. In the case of brain hyperactivity there is an increased number of connections between the neurons that are responsible for certain actions or creative ability.

Certain drugs work as inhibitors to disable those connections. In other words, the drug prevents the creation of some of those connections. It is unclear which connections exactly they act on and there are no clinical scientific proofs of effects on the creativity or other functions of the child if the drug were not taken.

In addition, it is not clear which new connections could have been created, or the short- and long-term effect.

In certain cases, the drug is given for the purpose of lowering the hyperactivity of the child, so s/he will cause no disturbance in class or at home.

We do not know if the use of such inhibitors means the loss of another Einstein.

Any new drug needs marketing and clinical research to prove its efficacy. Pharmaceutical companies employ physicians to assist them to this end.

Because of their particular relationship with powerful pharmaceutical companies, physicians prescribe certain drugs that are not necessarily appropriate, which can lead to conflicts of interest in certain cases.

The cooperation and collaboration between the education system and the supporting psychiatric field are criticized by those who claim that drugs are too readily prescribed. This raises the question of whether our children's interests are being best served.

Is the need for classroom silence parameter factor in the decision to drug our children?

Obviously, there are many cases where drugs are required.

There is a need, however, to check and seek second opinions about the need for specific medical treatment, the need for and the efficacy of the specific drug and its correct dosage. In addition to psychological and medical treatments, there are many supplementary remedies.

Not all have rational and scientific bases and the confusion is exploited by certain care providers for monetary gain.

Homeopathic treatments have been disputed and their efficacy is questionable, but if they relax children and their parents, then why not use them?

It is advisable, however, to consult the family physician first especially to avoid any undesirable drug interaction.

5. Parents, Children and Diagnosis.

CERTAIN PARENTS simply will not accept the diagnosis and the fact that their children need medical, psychological treatment or special education. They run between the experts and care providers, until they find a diagnosis they can live with or they think is the right one.

Those parents are inflicting unnecessary pressure on their children and family. The impression often given is that they require treatment more than their children.

The rate of false positives or misdiagnosis is too high. It is too high even if we take into account that sensitivity together with specificity is above 80%. If your child falls within the 20%, for you it is 100% misdiagnosis, unnecessary and sometimes harmful treatments, which may affect your child's entire future life.

Children with syndromes have different communication systems from the rest of the population. Therefore, someone is needed who can translate their needs into a language that adults can understand.

In psychometric and other tests, children with ADD and other syndromes may face an unfair situation compared with normal children in two respects.

One refers to the total time dedicated to the test and the other to the expected speed of responses to the questions.

In many cases children know the answer, but owing to the syndrome their concentration and response time may be longer than that allocated.

ADD and ADHD appear in boys about twice as much as in girls.

Why?

Is it because more boys are diagnosed or because behavioural disturbances are less observed in girls? Does the reason lie in genetics or hormones?

In the middle of the twentieth century, the number of daily tasks and external stimulation were fewer than those of today and they moved quite slowly on the timescale. This is obvious in the films from that era. Even the action movies were relatively slow, but had substantial text and dialogue.

Today tasks have evolved to multi-tasks; films are faster and contain more visual stimulation but less text and dialogue, except in the films of Woody Allen or Ingmar Bergman.

In today's society, whether it is democratic or not, the majority decides and expresses opinions, usually biased and loaded with prejudice, about who is exceptional or unacceptable. It starts with kindergarten and lasts throughout our entire life.

During the dark ages, we burned those deviants who looked odd, behaved irrationally or said strange and illogical things, like 'the earth is round'...

Galileo, Da Vinci and others were strange by normal standards.

It is hard to describe what our world would look like without them. We made their life difficult and in spite of that, they achieved excellence and innovation in the arts and sciences.

For certain children, many daily sounds are translated after a while into noise. For some of them it is difficult to cope with all that noise.

It is probable that the problem existed in the past but we failed to diagnose it, labelling such hyperactive children as naughty or slow.

The future entails more challenges and more noise, and there will be a need for children to face those challenges.

Many famous people like Edison, Mozart, Tesla, Dali and others were hyperactive. They were known for their unique temperament. They achieved greatness, perhaps because of rather than in spite of their attention deficit disorder. If the genes of ADD children have been selected or designed by nature for a new generation of creative inventors, then perhaps the phenomenon does not need treatment as much as refinement and acceptance.

By treating such children we inhibit evolution and progress and we reduce them to acceptable, average and normative levels.

Nature identified a need and it is trying to supply humanity with a new adaptable breed who will satisfy that need. They are the special *children of tomorrow*.

Accordingly, we should consider the qualifications and talents of those special children as a gift and not as a syndrome which needs psychological or medical treatment.

We need to support and encourage them to develop those talents and not inhibit them. Such children have grown up to be creative and passionate adults showing a significant decrease of the negative phenomena defined by the experts.

Verbal violence has no less a negative effect than physical violence and both should be eliminated. Parental insults, yelling and threats achieve nothing apart from discharging their frustration.

These situations cause the child to disconnect from his/her surroundings and withdraw into him/herself.

The child faces many difficulties at school and ought to feel that at his/her home s/he will be protected, understood and loved.

There is an obvious influence of family relationship on the condition and the functionality of the child. It should be emphasized that nobody is guilty in this situation. It is useless to blame parents or grandparents for bad genetics.

Not only is it incorrect, but it adds to the bad atmosphere that the child has to live in.

There is a significant difference and distance between children and parents, much more than in the past. It is probably the first time in human history that children have special skills that their parents lack, such as IT and other technological skills.

This knowledge gap generates disrespect and certain haughtiness in children, who are disappointed that their parents cannot operate a DVD or computer.

Our children are quick to comprehend, impatient and intolerant and will reject deviants.

It is true that children were cruel in the past to their eccentric friends, but these days their cruelty is amplified.

Today's children are quite superficial, searching for the easy, simple and immediate or instant.

Children born into the middle-upper class dedicate less thought to future economic and financial issues, and the consequence is a low common denominator and lack of effort to achieve for excellence.

The professional literature recommends a *strong father*, but not a violent one, who can generate proper parameters in terms of permitting and forbidding certain behaviours.

Here is a short list from those recommendations, about ideal parents for children with ADHD syndrome:

The boy has need of a strong and strict father.

*The father may be seen as 'ghost terrorífico' by
the boy, who may develop fear and hate,
but at the same time also love and respect.*

*The presence of a strong father is indispensable
so that the boy will be able to process the hatred
that inevitably he will feel toward someone.*

*The actual presence of the father at home is
indispensable to support the maternal authority
and to be constituted
as the representative of law and order.*

*The attitude of the mother is fundamental,
together with that of the father.*

A problem arises in cases when a significant difference between parental profiles is obvious.

The child suffers distress when s/he lives with a dominant father and with a weak mother or vice versa.

Psychologists require such parents to coordinate their positions and attitude.

The dominant parent will be required to adopt a lower profile and the weak parent a higher profile and be more assertive. When one of the parents is unable to perform that task, the situation may get worse.

There are cases where there is a gap between the parents in the permissive area.

This gap is usually generated by the mother, and the authoritative figure is usually the father. In such a case it is recommended that the father should stop being *responsible* for the *punishment* issues, which will lower his profile. It is essential, however, that at the same time the mother *increases* her profile and becomes more *assertive*.

In the past, problematic children were 'treated' with 'local punishment' by their parents and teachers. In Europe, they used to make children kneel on corn, hit their fingernails, slap their face and inflict other physical punishments on different body parts.

Parents used to accept these punishments, albeit with some reservations, and to support their understanding they sought reassurance from the Bible:

> He that spareth his rod hateth his son; but he that loveth him chasteneth him betimes (Proverbs 13:24).

This means that a father who does not discipline and punish his child is not educating him and therefore he does not love him.

Although the reference to 'son' is to the generic name for children, in this context boys are the subject. Punishing children using physical violence never solved anything; on the contrary, it only amplified the conflict and generated additional problems.

But…yes, there is a *but*…, society went from one radical extreme to another. Although today such punishment is legally forbidden, it still exists. We went from being punishing parents to being soft and over-protective.

Today's parents are spineless, and fail to set any limits, so that everything and anything goes. This does not reduce the level of violence but actually increases it.

What happened? Why are we a more violent society than in the past?

Obviously, there is no one simple answer to that question. One reason might be that we opened the door unwittingly and let the violence in.

We did it by misunderstanding our children, without establishing proper family relations and by ignoring their needs. We let them call us by our first name and not Dad or Mum, we became their friends, instead of keeping a proper distance.

We lost the discipline of the relationship we had with our own parents.

In the context of parents, the high divorce rate among the general population, and particularly among families with special children, should be mentioned as a factor affecting children with certain syndromes.

Parents in the past spent more quality time with their children. Research shows that today parents spend no more than fifteen minutes on average per day.

Because of their agonized consciousness of the difficulties, some parents became servants of their children and lost their dignity.

The education system in school faces many problems. There are no leadership, no rules, no discipline and no order. They have no solution to the increasing rate of violence. It should be emphasized that violence is not genetic, but it is acquired, and there are many ways to minimize it. Real-time online video surveillance with the awareness of the children can reduce violence at school. Such monitoring, even at the cost of privacy, is essential to document and monitor visitors and strangers in the school and surrounding area.

Drivers drive more carefully when the police are nearby.

We assume that children will behave better when they know that they are being watched.

There is a significant increase of alcohol usage between the ages of eleven and seventeen. There is no doubt that it is one of the reasons for the increase in violence.

The solution is similar to what Mayor Rudy Giuliani implemented in Manhattan, New York. He used 'zero tolerance', imposing immediate punishment, even for small crimes, and succeeded in significantly reducing New York's crime rate.

Alcohol and medication are a lethal combination. Special attention should be paid to those children who use alcohol and drive.

Investment in advertising at the national level, especially in schools, using audio-visual and real lectures, may assist in reducing both alcohol and violence levels. The campaign must include strong messages about the results of using alcohol and the punishment imposed if violence is used.

6. Treatment Within The Family.

Parents must seek support and cooperation from their own parents. The grandparents of the child are part of the rehabilitation and treatment process.

There is a need to verify that the child is not mistreated by the grandparents because of their ignorance of the situation.

Their cooperation is essential in carrying out the policy and the treatment recommended by the proper medical and psychological care providers.

Parents must explain the new situation to the other children in the family, give them specific tasks and obtain their cooperation in treating the sibling with the syndrome. It is vital to explain that their sibling is not sick, but needs help. S/he has unique qualifications in certain areas and lacks them in other areas. S/he needs their love and support, which s/he will reciprocate in future.

7. The Education System.

WE SEE an increasing gap between the relationships of children and the education system. The schools of today are quite archaic.

In most cases they have not followed the changing technology and the changing needs of modern children. This statement is supported by the archaic education methods and the outdated tools used. In the past, schools not only taught but educated as well. They were almost the only source of knowledge and information, and therefore it was impossible to criticize them or verify that the information taught was correct and up to date.

Today children have to sit quietly in one place, listening to the teacher's voice, which is sometimes quite loud and eventually becomes 'noise' in the brain of the special child.

On average, there are about three disturbed children in every classroom, some of whom have ADHD syndrome. Instead of removing or suspending them, another method is advised.

Collaborate with them, let them participate in class activity, give them the stage and flow with their needs. Usually, children who disturb in class send a message: 'I am bored'. This message is directed at the teacher. Teachers should identify the problem, i.e. why those children are not involved in class activities.

Often the solution is simple. They were teased or they simply did not understand the question or the situation; it is important to find out what bothers them. Removing those children from class may help temporarily but the problem is not resolved but often intensified. By removing children from class, teachers signal to the other students that they have marked those children as problematic and they will treat them accordingly. Yet if teachers succeed in persuading them to cooperate, they will benefit from that as well.

They might become better and more acceptable teachers admired and appreciated by the students, the school and especially by the parents.

Teachers are recommended to develop good relationships and cooperation with parents.

This is important in general, but particularly in cases involving children with ADHD or other syndromes.

In the regular education system, teachers do not have the patience and some of them lack the qualifications required to deal with such children. Empathy and cooperation between teachers and parents in certain cases may eliminate the need to transfer the child to the special education system.

8. IMAGINARY FRIENDS.

IMAGINARY FRIENDS are part of a normative evolutionary phase which gives the child an efficient platform to express him/herself, usually in a very creative way. Most children have imaginary friends at some point in their early life.

Those friends will eventually disappear. They disappear simply because with time the child loses interest.

For some children, the imaginary friend may appear in the form of an animal, such as an elephant, tiger or dog.

The child believes that the imaginary friend will fulfil his/her wishes and believes that the friend is a kind of 'super-friend'. This friend is very efficient and effective in the child's life and may have many goals. It may help in facing and coping with feelings that are difficult to express.

Sometimes, those feelings are negative in nature.

When the child is angry and wants to react with violence, s/he is aware that it is forbidden, and then the imaginary friend comes to help.

All negative feelings and wrongdoings are transferred to the imaginary friend: 'I did not do it' or 'He did it'.

Because the imaginary friend was created by the child, s/he feels safer and relaxes with it and the communication between them solves many problems, including loneliness and boredom.

The friend eases the child's pain, anxiety and fear and, as mentioned earlier, eventually he will disappear.

It is important to remember that the imaginary friend will not replace real friends.

9. LOVING TREATMENT.

*What cannot be resolved with love
can be resolved with more love (Author)*

MUCH HAS BEEN WRITTEN ABOUT LOVE and there is no need to repeat here the words of the world's great philosophers, lovers and poets.

It could be quite disappointing to analyse falling in love from the scientific perspective. If you were told that it was all to do with a very small area of the brain and a transient chemical process, it could well kill desire and the longing for love.

The psychologist Robert Sternberg defined love in the context of an interpersonal relationship as a combination of three elements: *intimacy*, *commitment* and *passion*.

Baruch de Spinoza, the seventeenth-century philosopher, identified three different elements defining love: *desire*, *joy* and *sorrow*.

There are no conditions in love, no *if, but* or *when*. Sometimes love is painful, disappointing and makes us lose our head.

Love is a function of age. Romeo and Juliet's teenage love is not the same as adult love. The attitude to the word *love* and its significance is different not only in certain age groups, but also in different cultures.

We tend to associate the word *love* not only with humans but also with animals, items, food, behaviour and films.

Obviously, there is parental-family love, love of friends, love of neighbours and of course love of God (Leviticus 19:18):

Thou shalt love thy neighbour as thyself

If, however, *thyself* is narcissistic, it might be a destructive love. On the other hand, if it is a healthy narcissism, it might be a positive and interesting type of love. There are many types and groups of narcissistic behaviour defined and classified according to the amount of self-love involved.

According to Freud, our ego develops during infancy and therefore we do not possess the knowledge of self-love at birth. Later in life, our parents, friends and social environment mould our image of the aspired self, which builds and generates our ego.

There is nothing wrong with mild narcissism or mild ego. An egoistic couple can be quite happy. Even Freud realized that exclusive self-love might not be as abnormal as previously thought.

Narcissus was a handsome Greek youth, according to the myth, who fell in love with his reflection in a pool when he saw it for the first time. He died when he realized that he was unable to consummate his love. The narcissus flower bears his name.

Love brings more love.

Love is a rare and precious thing. If you are among the lucky ones, you must do everything, but everything, to preserve it.

10. ALTERNATIVE METHODOLOGY.

THE FOLLOWING METHODOLOGY may be applicable not only for ADHD cases, but also for cerebral palsy, deafness etc., where communication or the lack of it is a dominant factor in the treatment process.

The proposed treatment and methodology principally involve the inner family circle, where we all have ability to implement the recommended changes. The regimen sits apart from the conventional methods, which constitute a kind of general formula applied to diverse classified groups as a collective treatment.

Assuming that you the reader have somebody in your family with a syndrome and you wish to assist and get involved in learning how to treat and improve life for that child and his/her family. The subjects described here will enrich your tool-box and will enable you to tailor the treatment to your case.

The recommendations made here as part of the proposed treatment must be seen as a complementary activity to the diverse treatments proposed and implemented by qualified experts in the field.

It is important to perform the diagnosis as early as possible, when irregular behaviour is observed either by the parents or by the education system.

In order to understand the special situation that your child is in, imagine that you are transferred to a parallel universe, where you do not understand the local language.

You are in your own house, surrounded by a worried family, everybody is crying. You are lying in bed; you do not understand what's going on. You are shouting, but your voice is not heard, you want to move, but you are paralysed. You are in a nightmare and totally helpless.

Less dramatically... you are in a class surrounded by children. You are the same age as your child, but the other children speak a language which you do not understand.

Your entire communicative ability is limited to touching...

In a short time you will be outcast, labelled and alone. In your mind you are fully aware of the surrounding situation, but you are unable to communicate properly.

This scenario is similar to the situation your child is in. They need to learn and adopt the proper communication skills.

Some children will use physical contact, some will try to attract attention by shouting and cursing and some will simply disconnect, give up and leave the class or the house.

The following actions may assist you to understand better and become closer to your special child. First, get acquainted with your child, without any prejudice. Try to ignore what was said, diagnosed and labelled by all professionals and others. Invest quality time and monitor your child's activities closely. Find the things they like and do not like in all areas: food, play, school, study, friends, etc.

This information is critical if you are to arrive at the right treatment.

When a child loves and enjoys a specific activity, positive and efficient communication exists during that time. Use that time to merge or to insert messages and desired behaviours that you would like the child to adopt, improve, or correct, without interfering or disturbing the specific activity. The child will not communicate well when s/he is required to do certain tasks against his/her will.

If forced to do it, usually s/he will cooperate, but without any enthusiasm. This is not a good time to educate or send corrective messages.

Let us assume that the child is particularly fond of the image of Tom the cat (from the *Tom and Jerry* TV programme). S/he will be more open to receiving messages from a puppet in the shape of Tom than from a parent. There are many suitable interactive programmes and a list should be available from your therapist or on the internet.

11. Food, Sleep And Noise.

FOOD HAS a significant effect on the level of attention disorder. Therefore, it is vital to monitor your child's diet. It is sensible to avoid junk food, preservatives, edible colours or over-indulgence in snacks and sweets.

You should be aware that most cereals comprise over 30% sugar. Although sugar's influence on ADHD is a controversial subject, it is currently recommended to avoid excessive usage.

It is important to provide a proper breakfast containing proteins and carbohydrates such as whole-wheat bread and egg. Right nourishment at the right time of the day is important, especially for those who are on medication.

It is important to eat before taking the medication, especially Ritalin, which causes loss of appetite inter alia.

Proper and timely sleep has an influence on the child's functioning and behaviour. Therefore, a routine sleep of at least eight hours is desirable, as is sleeping at fixed regular hours and not after 22:00.

Special children have a hearing capability and sensitivity to noise above the average and most of them like music. Therefore, it is important to facilitate a quiet and relaxed atmosphere.

Do not do – Do not yell, insult, curse. Do not be judgmental and never raise your hand to a child.

Do – Love, hug, encourage, support, forgive, understand, smile, and love more.

You should award and encourage a child for good behaviour and revoke certain rights for inappropriate behaviour.

You have to explain to the child the basic law of physics:

For every action there is a reaction.

Therefore, 'If you won't eat, you'll be hungry', 'If you hurt your friend, sister or your brother, they will feel pain, suffer, and they will not be your friend and will not play with you', 'If you don't shower, you'll smell and your friends will avoid you'.

It is important to respond immediately to any violent expression and monitor closely what is going on at school. Whether your child is the abusee or the abuser, you need to respond and treat the problem from the first with 'zero tolerance' Participate in parent-teacher meetings to resolve disputes between children. Without immediate and proper intervention, the situation might get worse.

If the child is on medication, it is vital to look for possible side-effects and report them to the family physician. Many drugs are addictive and the right dosage is no less important than the right medication.

If you observe anger outbreaks, and the child is constantly tired and difficult to talk to, it is important to check the medication and its dosage.

When you see that your child is capable and enjoys doing a, b or c, but does not like or is unwilling to do d, e or f, you should focus on a, b or c, and compliment and encourage the child. Later you can teach him/her slowly, step by step, d, e or f, but try to get some cooperation and do not force the pace. You should avoid 'angry prophesies' such as: 'If you do not...then you'll be this and that'. In general, do not send negative messages or generate negative energy.

Your child is in a difficult phase in his/her life. S/he is fighting to be accepted as 'cool' at school and at home s/he expects warmth, love and support.

When s/he has to listen to 'prophesy speeches' too often s/he may give up and submit to despair.

Sometimes, a prophesy is self-fulfilling. When a label or certain adjective is used, the child may adopt it, even if s/he does not necessarily deserve it. S/he may say to him/herself: 'If I am expected to be...then why should I try being something else?'

It is advisable to teach the child to take care of him/herself. Yes, it sounds unrealistic, but it is possible.

First, show him/her, in a video for example, another child who looks like him/her and has a similar background. That child will carry out certain tasks, and will talk about and explain them in a way that your child can understand and relate to.

An alternative might be to video-record the child unawares and show him/her later. You can explain that this is how s/he behaved, said or did and together you can find what was wrong and what would be the right way the next time.

The process of training the child in diverse simulations of situations will persuade him/her that there are other ways of self-expression. Accordingly, step by step s/he might change his/her pattern of behaviour and adopt a more acceptable one. Physical activities such as judo, horse riding and the like are strongly recommended.

Such organized group or individual activities may enable the child to divert their extra energies and release them at a suitable place and time.

The child may adopt rules and disciplines through appropriate activities, self-organization, persistence and the carrying out of certain tasks.

In addition, it is desirable to organize literary activities, such as discussions about books, poems or songs, which may assist the acquisition of self-confidence. In general, special children do not like change. Therefore, you should prepare a weekly schedule, which is more or less filled with known, fixed and mutually agreed activities. Children are quite conservative and will not try new things willingly.

For example, usually they will refuse to eat new and different food.

In this context and in general, it is recommended to adopt the following attitude or rule: 'You don't have to eat it, but you have to taste and try it'.

This approach is applicable to many contexts; it will encourage curiosity and experience of new things, but it should not be enforced.

In terms of negotiations, what is good for adults is also good for children. We as parents should emphasize the areas and the subjects where we have agreement and mutual interests.

12. Parental Involvement.

We should use our parental authority to emphasize the rationale and logic behind our demands, without forgetting the benefits, namely, the reward for cooperating or the consequences of disagreement and unwillingness to cooperate.

The following practical advice is aimed at parents of special children.

Keep your promises and do not make any if you have no intention of keeping them. Tell your children about your childhood. Spend quality time with them as often as you can. Be an example and a role model to your children. Take holidays, go on trips and spend time on a one-on-one basis.

Tell them stories; they will remember your voice more than the content of the stories.

Take them to your workplace. Get to know their friends. Always listen to them.

Make a kite and fly it together. Define consistent rules and limits.

Take them to museums, zoos and other fun places. Make them participate in home tasks and various assignments. Most importantly, show empathy, warmth and lots of love.

Parents have different styles: permissive, dominant, authoritative, indifferent or even, sadly, neglectful and abusive.

The desired style is an efficient attitude which enables one to find a balance between respect and consideration for the child's need and parental expectations.

There should be a balance between excessive parental presence and the lack of it. We should provide enough freedom and privacy and at the same time monitor and supervise the child's activities.

During adolescence the child goes through many changes. Those changes are emotional, physical and social, all in a relatively short time.

This is a difficult period not only for the child, but for the parents as well. Parental authority is questioned and power struggles are quite common.

Parents should learn to handle conflicts and confrontation wisely, decisively and with lots of love and understanding.

You should adopt a reciprocal basis of give & take and reward & punishment and let the child win some arguments as well.

Parents should set clear consistent standards and be a role model to follow. Standards should be such that parents themselves can stand by them and follow them.

You cannot expect total agreement on all objects of dispute. As in any other conflict, you may insert certain 'fake' demands for the purpose of removing them at a later stage.

A conflict will be positively terminated when both sides feel they have won. When we set demands and standards to follow, there is a need to respond properly when they are not followed or are violated.

Specific standards are culture-oriented and might be problematic, especially in a multi-cultural but highly segregated society.

The activation and implementation of parental authority is essential for the proper evolution of the adolescent child and is particularly important for the special child.

If the child is experiencing a difficult day, if s/he was bullied at school or just in a bad mood, which is a common situation, try the following experiment.

Draw a circle of about one inch diameter and blacken it on an A4 sheet of white paper.

Put the page in front of the child's eyes and ask: 'What do you see?'.

The usual response is: 'A black circle'. Move the page a few feet away and ask: 'What has happened to the big black circle?' 'It became a small point': at greater distance the point is barely visible.

Explain to the child that when the big black circle is close to his/her eyes, it is equivalent to his/her current feelings, namely, everything looks black and gloomy. But in time it will become a small point, which will disappear and all will be white and clean.

Special children are more visually than textually oriented; therefore such a metaphor might be accepted and understood better than verbal explanations and encouragement, which should be given in any case.

Children at school have always picked on the weak, the odd and the different. It is a cruel reality, even in the animal world. They make fun of others, ostracise them and sometimes even use physical violence.

Your child is in a difficult situation.

If s/he responds with violence, s/he might be expelled from school.

If s/he does nothing, s/he might become the butt of the class. There are no magical solutions, but you can minimize the bullying scenarios by using the following process.

Summon as soon as possible after the event a meeting under school's auspices with the parents of the bullying child and parents of other children involved. It is important to prepare the parents before the meeting in order to minimize the possibility of any dispute.

It should be made clear to the bullying child's parents that lack of cooperation on their part might cause their child to be expelled from school.

The meeting could be held on school premises, but it is better to select a neutral place like a garden or a park or somewhere without external disturbances.

Sometimes, one meeting is enough to show the children involved that their parents are cooperating and share a mutual interest in resolving the situation.

Moreover, the children must see a united front on the part of parents and school. They should realize that they unanimously present acceptable, expected and desired normative behaviour. The special child should be taught not to raise his/her hand, but at the same time not to run away. S/he can confront the bullying child face to face, tell him/her that s/he will not tolerate abuse, s/he does not expect such behaviour from a classmate and if it continues s/he will be forced to report it to the teacher and parents.

Such confrontation sends the bullying child a message, 'I am not afraid of you', which may cause him/her to think twice.

You are sitting in your car. What are all the options open to you? Move forward, backward, left, right. Yet there is one more option, which is to stay where you are.

Teach your children that when they are faced with choosing between a or b, they always have a third option, namely not to choose or not to decide now. 'I'll think about it', 'I'll consult with my parents and choose later' should be their response.

In life there is more than one option, regardless of what others may wish us to do.

Children make many decisions every day. Some of them are normative and others are a response to threats made by hostile classmates or other children: for example, 'You have two options, either you give me your sandwich or I'll hurt you'. You should teach your child that s/he has more options when s/he is given two bad choices.

I mentioned earlier the law of physics governing action and reaction. In this case, the robbed child could respond: 'If you eat my sandwich, I'll be hungry and I'll have to inform my parents, who will call your parents', 'If you hurt me, I'll suffer pain and I'll be forced to report it', 'I have an idea; today, we will share my sandwich and tomorrow we will share yours'.

A stronger child might respond: 'I have no intention of giving you my sandwich, and about hurting me, well, you know what the result will be'. If you are the bullying child's parents, do not use any punishment, because it might only make the situation worse. Invite the other child for a joint picnic.

Try to connect and not separate children. Explain to your child the consequences which all of you will have to suffer if s/he does not behave. There are parents who still say: 'If he is hurting you, be a man, hurt him back'. This attitude not only will not resolve the conflict, but in most cases it will enhance it. Violence triggers more violence.

The phenomenon of bullying and violence is much less common in the special education system.

One of the reasons may be because there are fewer violent interactions between children at special schools. The qualified teacher will handle any outburst of violence immediately, firmly and sensitively.

Violence is an outburst of energy without control and aim. It is a waste of energy, inefficient and useless. Therefore, we have to channel our children's energy positively. There is no point in suppression and punishment in such cases and education on the right use of such energy must start at an early age.

A punishing parent is a powerless and weak parent.

This parent has no practical solution and the only response s/he can make is to demonstrate his/her parental authority by applying punishment.

Many parents respond with a negative attitude: 'Don't go there' or 'Don't do that'.

They tend to emphasize 'what not to do' and not 'what to do', which is the preferred positive attitude.

We have to teach our children to take responsibility for their actions and not let them blackmail us emotionally.

They can do it with some success as they are aware of its effect and realize that it works. A positive and a rewarding daily interaction system between us and our children should be developed. We have to show involvement as well as supervision and reward good behaviour with compliments, without generating a link between a child's achievement or success and monetary or material compensation.

It is preferable to say to a child 'You succeeded because you have invested a lot of time and effort in preparing your homework' rather than 'You succeeded because you are smart'. The latter sentence sends the message 'I am smart, therefore I don't need to make an effort to study', whereas the conclusion to be inferred from the former sentence is 'I succeeded because I have invested' and this will teach the child that in order to succeed s/he first has to invest effort.

In the case of failure, there is a need to encourage children in a positive way and explain that: 'It is OK and normal to fail occasionally, it is part of life' and the question is how to face and cope with failure and rejection. Teaching children to strive for excellence is good but at the same time it is important to prepare them for occasional failures as well, to encourage them to 'climb back on the horse' in case of a fall or failure. Success after failure is satisfying and will strengthen the child, who may learn from it for the future.

It is important to emphasize that the aim here was to generate stimulation to find creative ways to assist ourselves and our children to enjoy better communication and a better life together as a family.

13. THE POWER OF BELIEF.

BELIEF IS A BASIC HUMAN RIGHT. We humans have a need to believe. Sometimes, that need has a power of its own and we follow it without the ability to stop, avoid it or ignore it.

When we talk about belief most of us think immediately about religion and faith, but belief is much more than that. In fact, faith is merely a subset forming part of a wider concept of belief.

It is true that religion is the common concept relating to belief and without it religion would not exist, but belief is a powerful energy that drives us to perform or to avoid many activities.

Belief cannot dwell in a realistic realm. Where there are facts and evidence, belief has no true basis for existence.

Faith and belief may exist in a world where reality, facts and evidence are replaced by personal emotions and irrational views or observations of things.

Sometimes factual events or archaeological findings or other material proofs can be ignored by a blind and fanatical believer. Such a person is unwilling to consider the possibility that their and their ancestors' belief may be irrational or based on an imaginative or speculative scenario.

Faith relies upon its believers. Believers in a common faith are united under its umbrella.

Faiths have historically used force to persuade and make people believe, in order to increase their membership.

Religion and science have a 'love-hate' relationship. Science is based and relies on proofs, reason, empirical evidence and rationalism.

Religion is based on faith and sometimes blind belief in a non-real or non-existing entity, belief in revelation and sacredness. For the believer, however, that entity may exist and be very real.

We could say that both religion and science are pursuing and seeking knowledge, albeit from a different perspective.

Human history and philosophy suggest, however, that science and religion are more in conflict than in agreement.

The search for a link or correlation between spirituality and neural phenomena is known as spiritual neuroscience or neuro-theology. Spiritual or religious experiences can be explained by neuro-theology and scientific neurological brain research findings.

Certain religious activities or beliefs can be associated with temporal lobe epilepsy seizures, during which an enhanced emotional response to religious words may be observed.

This finding indicates that the medial temporal lobe might be involved in generating some of the emotional reactions associated with religious stimulation.

Belief is fostered in many ways. Faith-related belief is usually maintained for a long period, or even a lifetime, if taught in early childhood.

Belief can be adopted if a person is influenced by a charismatic 'guru' or preacher.

Other types of belief may depend on the local community, tribe or country that one belongs to. We may adopt or change our beliefs when we are exposed to certain emotions, such as sexual implicated advertisements.

The power of advertisements, particularly those with sexual implications, can lead us to adopt new beliefs and habits, whether as consumers or as believers (in certain events, or in certain people, such as politicians...). We may be influenced by certain traumas, especially brain-related injury or disease.

Belief is originated and 'cooked' in our brain. Our thoughts are very powerful, whether positive or negative.

Accordingly, the power of belief has a tremendous influence on our life.

Recognition of this fact should mean we try to control and master our thoughts. The problem is that when emotions are involved negative thoughts and beliefs are all too common.

Can we modify and change our beliefs?

The answer to that question is yes.

Belief from a historical perspective is a human evolutionary process.

The more knowledge and experience we accumulate, the more tools we have and the greater our capabilities to change and modify our beliefs.

There are many ways to effect change but we have to assist in the process by doing things in a different manner.

Each person can develop a method in their own way. If we realize that our belief is limiting us or is a barrier to certain goals or achievements, we have to try to remove those obstacles by acting without hesitation or fear of failure.

If we want something or want to become a different person, we should act or simulate the scenario as if we have that thing or as if we are already that person we want to be.

If we do not believe that we can do it, then probably we will fail.

We have to overcome the fear of failure, which is the limiting factor.

We will be able to control the power of belief by training ourselves to think positively, acting and behaving as though we have already achieved our goals. We have to believe in our ability to make that change.

The power of belief states that: 'We can be whatever we *want* to be or whatever we *believe* we can be'.

Belief in clinical environment has a substantial impact on ill and injured patients. There are many cases of 'miraculous' recovery after cancer or crippling accident.

14. Biofeedback.

Biofeedback as used in neuroscience has shown cases where changing the patient's belief relieved or even cured the diagnosed complaint. This is a remarkable situation, whereby the patient may cure him/herself, if s/he is strong enough to believe that it is possible.

Placebo effect is another clinical area where the power of belief is obvious and has been proven to have a real impact on patient recovery. Patients are given a *real* drug or a *false* (placebo) drug treatment. The placebo phenomenon is that they do not know this and accordingly *believe* that they are getting a real and effective drug, which will improve or cure their illness. Thus believing is healing, the true power of belief.

From this phenomenon it follows that if we are cured by a fake drug then our belief could be applied successfully in other areas of our lives.

If we, or more precisely our brain, can be tricked like this, then we should apply the trick to boost self-esteem and belief in ourselves and in our abilities to overcome the many obstacles that life presents us with. Possibility to love presents a similar method of belief: 'Fake it till you make it'.

Our immune system is built to protect us from many external threats; however it fails when emotion and stress are involved.

If we permit 'bad energy' to enter our brain, we are flooded by bad emotions that can affect our physical body. This is the negative power of belief. The link of mind-spirit and body is obvious. We should realize that the power of belief can also work against us and may be a destructive force.

Therefore, we should avoid negativism and seek positivism. Above all, we have to believe in ourselves.

15. WILLPOWER.

WILLPOWER IS one of the significant human driving forces. We know that there is a power in our will, as in the saying: 'Where there is a will, there is a way'.

This willpower helps us to overcome the many difficulties and obstacles in our life. It is one of the major components needed for success.

The question is whether willpower is the same as free will. Free will can be defined as the act of choosing without any constraints. By choosing, I mean acting or thinking freely and independently.

Constraints can be classified into several groups of influence: psychological, social, physical, medical, ethical or other influences that might affect our will. In addition, our will may be linked to and dependent upon other factors such as religion, science or ethics. In neuroscience, for example, free will can help to explain human behaviour.

The existence of free will, however, is debated by philosophers rather than scientists.

In studying the brain, we can see in real time under MRI (magnetic resonance imaging), the process of decision-making. When we wish to move our hand, the brain sends the appropriate signal.

The question is this: 'Is there a time gap between the instant the decision was made and the time when the actual signal was sent?'.

Recent studies show that there is a time that could be as much as half a second or more. This finding shows that the brain makes a decision some time before we are aware of it, implying that we do not have free will.

This scientific finding may force us to redefine the concept of free will.

16. The Desire To Live.

A COMMON PHENOMENON is that when one half of a couple that has been together for a long time dies, the other also dies shortly afterwards. The usual, romantic, explanation is that they loved each other so much that they could not live without each other.

He or she died from a 'broken heart', 'could not live alone', 'was dependent on their spouse'.

Is there a correlation between the death of one spouse and the subsequent death of the other shortly afterwards?

The hypothesis is that the desire to live may have a certain effect on the immune system. The brain that is in control of our body may have a shut-down mechanism, which is activated in certain cases.

Those cases are similar to fatal accidents or certain illnesses, where the brain knows that it will not be able to cope. This mechanism may control 'suicide cells'.

In recent years, suicide cells or what scientists define as programmed cell death (PCD) has formed the basis for ongoing biogenetic research.

PCD is the death of a cell which is mediated by an intracellular programme.

There are three major types of PCDs. Type I cell death is called apoptosis. Type II is autophagic and Type III is necrotic cell-death. Cells can be killed by injurious agents or be instructed to commit suicide. If there is a threat to the integrity of an organism by certain cells, PCD is needed to destroy those cells.

Typical examples of such cases are: cells that are infected by viruses, DNA damage, cells of the immune system and cancer cells.

In certain types of cancer cells apoptosis is triggered by radiation or chemicals used for therapy.

What makes a cell decide to commit suicide?

The author believes that it is the imbalance between positive and negative signals sent by the brain.

If there is a lack of the positive signals (no desire to live) needed for survival and/or negative signals are sent meaning 'no desire to continue to live', the shut-down mechanism may be activated.

There have been numerous reports of cases where patients recovered miraculously after clearly being diagnosed with cancer. This phenomenon may be explained by the activation of the PCD mechanism by 'desire to live' positive signals.

In some cases, viruses that are associated with cancers may use tricks, like producing a protein that inactivates the apoptosis signal. In such cases the cancer cells will not only continue to live and proliferate, but they will become more resistant to apoptosis.

Further understanding of those tricks and decoy molecules generated to protect cancer cells would enable researchers to reactivate and overcome those protective tricks in order to destroy dangerous cancer cells.

The author also believes that future research on destroying and removing cancerous cells might be implemented in two phases.

The first phase would be to distinguish, mark and identify cancerous cells.

In phase two the target would be to activate suicide cells in the selected area or group of cells and bypass the existing protection of the cancer cells.

Strong psychological and family support is essential for such a recovery.

In addition, the patient must believe in and hope for a healthy and bright future.

17. NEUROPHILOSPHY AND EDUCATION.

NEUROPHILOSOPHY AND EDUCATION are an interesting and a promising area of research in terms of the interaction and relationship between educators and students.

On the one hand, we have the educator-teacher, who has knowledge and the experience on certain subjects and may be perceived as the 'transmitter'.

On the other, we have the student, who has the need to be educated. S/he needs or wishes to acquire knowledge for diverse purposes, such as an academic degree for professional use. The student may be perceived as the 'receiver'.

Actually, the process of learning-studying is a neuro-interaction between two brains, an indirect transmission using language as the medium of communication.

This process uses brain-language-sound generated on the transmitter side and brain-language-ears on the receiver side.

The receiver needs to translate, process and store the message in his/her brain. As this process is indirect between the two brains and involves several elements and organs, it is exposed to 'noise' and interference.

One such example is ADHD. There are other interfering elements in this process and the ability to receive the same transmission in a class environment varies from student to student.

Willingness to learn is a major factor in the student's ability to acquire the desired knowledge transmitted by the teacher. The student needs to open his/her receptors and receive the information in a certain form commensurate with his/her ability to understand.

The teacher must be in a transmitting mode and at the same time the student must be in a receiving mode. If the student is not in the receiving mode, the teacher's responsibility is to generate the appropriate conditions so that his/her messages will be properly received, at least by most students.

This type of education is more student-oriented, unlike the standard 'fit-all' methods.

If the receiver-student has receiving problems, the transmission and the transmitter must be checked. The ability to receive an unclear or encoded transmission depends on the receiving brain and its ability to decipher, analyse and store the message.

It is, however, primarily dependent on the quality, clarity and authenticity of the message transmitted by the teacher.

Understanding occurs when the receiver signals the transmitter, 'I have got it'. This acknowledgement can take many forms, such as a written or oral test, when the teacher can assess the student's understanding.

So how are those messages stored by the brain? Are all those messages stored in one location in our memory brain?

We do not yet know the answer but we know from neuro-imaging experiments that this process is neuron-dependent. We can observe 'action' or 'light-up' of our synapses during the learning process.

This fact suggests that information is not stored at one specific location but spread over a wider area of neurons. Another supporting fact is the ability of a patient suffering from post-traumatic brain injury or loss of certain parts of the brain to recover.

If that information was stored in one location only, such recovery would be impossible.

In addition, we know that our memory is associative, which means that we can recall certain scenarios or information from our 'experience' data base memory by using related and unrelated triggers, such as sound, smell, touch or other visual or audio experiences.

This proves that there are many interconnections in the same cluster of data to be retrieved.

The recall process enhances and strengthens the neuro-connections between the relevant cells, which accordingly will keep the data stored viable, accessible and fresh.

Learning will generate similar enrichment of the neurons and their interconnections.

Our brain consists of trillions of neurons, with a huge number of complex interconnections. What differ from brain-to-brain are the types of neurons and the specific neurochemical interaction among the neurons.

It is interesting to note that the structure of clusters of neurons and their specific interconnections may have an effect on one's ability to learn and an influence on speed of understanding and reaction time to intellectual stimulations.

At birth, our brain is very plastic, that is, its capability to process and store sensory information is very high.

Neuronal connections are generated, broken and regenerated, which suggests that early educational and environmental stimulations are essential for the child's evolution.

This is the critical period of the development of the child's linguistic, cognitive and social abilities.

A classical question is whether the infant brain is empty, a tabula rasa, at birth. The Greek philosopher Aristotle (fourth century B.C.E.) was probably the first to introduce the tabula rasa (blank slate) idea.

According to the tabula rasa theory, an infant's brain is empty of mental content, which will be acquired later with experience and perception. Although the 'tools' or the brain cells are already formed at birth, only after gaining experience will we see the generation of neurons' inter-connections.

As Aristotle and subsequent supporters of his theory were not privy to recent genetic discoveries, the tabula rasa theory may not be applicable or accepted as a deterministic valid concept.

Today it is believed that a child's cerebral cortex is pre-programmed to enable the processing of sensory input, emotions and environmental stimulations.

The author does not support the tabula-rasa theory and he believes that there are genetically transferred data or imprints.

Those genetic imprints may have a clear impact and influence on the child's behaviour and even on its brain's ability to process and store information.

Technological evolution is still happening in computer technology, when we communicate with computers not only via a keyboard, mouse or touch-screen, but also via sound or voice.

Similar evolution is happening in medicine such as brain-activated devices based on EEG (electro-encephalo-graphs).

In future we could experience direct brain-to-brain transmission similar to telepathy.

Telepathy derives from the Greek ('distant experience') and it is a kind of mental transfer from one brain to another.

As it is not a clearly reproducible phenomenon, the scientific community has not reached consensus.

Telepathy is well accepted, however, albeit largely used in science fiction.

As many science fiction scenarios became reality in time, however, the author believes that some brain-to-brain communication will be possible in future.

Neuro-imaging is one of the scientific areas where this type of communication is being researched and interesting results are anticipated.

The conclusion is that educational methods must correspond and comply with our brain function and its ability to store information and not on a dogmatic rigorous unified system as exemplified in most schools.

18. GLOBAL EDUCATION METHODS.

GLOBAL EDUCATION METHODS are generally intended to transfer specific knowledge or skills developed by a country or educational authority to a general collective audience of students, but different students accept, absorb and understand or fail to understand the same material in very different ways. These differences may be explained by multiple factors which affect students during lessons.

Learning may be impeded by cultural, ethnic or linguistic barriers, as well as personal psychological factor such as mood, fatigue and lack of attention.

These factors can affect the learning of the typical student, and it may take extra effort to understand the material being presented. Students with ADD find learning tasks significantly more difficult and should be taught using different methods.

The two major brain capabilities involved in learning are memory and understanding. Whilst it might appear that these two capabilities are interdependent this is a misconception.

I would like to argue that it is possible to have a very good memory without understanding, but that good understanding is not possible without memory.

Moreover, to succeed in certain academic spheres one needs to be highly capable of both memory and understanding.

This can be illustrated by considering the differences between the capabilities required to succeed in humanities subjects and sciences.

An excellent memory may be a necessary and a sufficient condition for success in the humanities, but whilst it is a necessary condition for success in the sciences, it is not sufficient; in the sciences understanding is crucial to success.

More specifically, a student will be able to pass an examination in history provided that he or she has learned the text and remembers it, whereas to pass an examination in mathematics the student must understand the material as well as remembering it. A good memory is not enough to solve mathematics problems.

All students develop their own method for remembering and understanding material which is presented to them.

There are individual differences in the conditions required to support learning. Some prefer to study in the evening, in a quiet atmosphere, with a cup of tea or coffee to hand, whereas others can study at any time, and in any place, with loud music in the background.

An individual's learning is affected by his or her physical and mental status, including factors such as hunger, fatigue, stress, headaches, social and personal problems to name but a few.

Most of us succeed in overcoming the variety of obstacles that we face and finish our studies. Success or failure in studies can be attributed to a large number of potential disrupters of learning.

Throughout the world there are private educational institutes, some of which are supported by local community organisations or religious organisations.

When the government is not supporting those institutes financially, there is no real oversight of the curriculum or teaching in these educational institutes.

Obviously, these institutes have a specific educational agenda and do not necessarily follow mainstream educational methods.

Religious organisations focus on self-preservation and are therefore interested in maintaining or increasing membership. Similarly terrorist organisations want to educate young children to support their cause. Their programme may contain certain psychological elements such as brain-washing propaganda.

Both religious and terrorist organisations may censor the information to which students have access and feed them disinformation when it suits their purpose. Such educational strategies are vital to their survival.

If we could look in on a typical classroom about a century ago, we would see that there were very limited tools and media available to teachers. We would see a limited numbers of books, a blackboard and chalks, pencils, a small number of fountain pens with inkwells. The classroom would get very cold in winter and too hot in summer and students of a wide range of ages would study in one class; sometimes boys and girls would have to study in different classrooms. There would be a very strict, rather aggressive teacher, with a stick and almost unlimited authority to punish the students.

Today teachers have access to a wide range of tools and media such as television, computers, the Internet, films, theatre, art, a wide range of books and unlimited online access to a vast body of information.

Most educational establishments have air-conditioned classrooms and boys and girls of the same age are taught together by patient teachers with very limited means and authority to punish. The advent of new, open and uncontrolled media has meant that global education systems now have the problem that there is too much information readily available to anyone of any age.

Young children can be exposed to free pornography via the Internet if there is a lack of parental control or supervision and this may distort their understanding of sexuality.

The global education system changed radically in the last century and so have the students, who are now very knowledgeable and smart.

They are aware of their rights and in most cases have more control over their education than has the system. Education systems throughout the world should also enable students with special needs to study in an appropriate environment.

19. Tomorrow's Teachers.

Tomorrow's teachers should realise the importance of making cross-cultural connections in classroom, where it will still be important to establish authority and develop a good relationship with the students as well as promoting appropriate relationships among students.

In the broad sense education since the time of creation can be defined as a learning process by which a group of people transfer their experience, accumulated knowledge, values and beliefs to the next generation. Education may also include autodidactic learning and any experience which affects how an individual feels, thinks and acts.

To date formal education has been divided into stages, which may include preschool education, primary and secondary education, university education and other forms of higher education.

Acquiring knowledge involves cognitive processes such as communication, perception, observation and reasoning.

These processes are characteristic of humanity. We are all aware that with time the thirst for knowledge is increasing.

The future of humanity is closely tied to advances in technology. Education is a function of technology, amongst other factors, and so it is inevitable that people who are excluded from technological progress for any reason will be penalised educationally.

Some of the factors directly or indirectly related to education which can significantly affect our way of life are lack of information or a surplus of information, stubbornness, stupidity, vanity and arrogance. They can affect our success in both personal and professional domains, causing us to miss opportunities.

Technological developments in social networking such as Facebook have opened up exciting, new educational opportunities worldwide.

Platforms such as Facebook offer educators the opportunity to combine social networking with global education methods and systems.

Teachers, schools and other educational organisations throughout the world could exploit these new social technological applications for educational innovation.

Since World War II there has been a growing need for school buildings. The shortage of classroom space is a heavy burden on governments and educational systems across the world. Some people claim that the lack of dedicated learning spaces can be resolved by providing a wide range of resources in the formal and non-formal education sectors in order to make education available to the least privileged sections of our society.

These resources may include e-learning and online education.

An interesting study indicated that on average students in an online learning environment performed better than those studying in face-to-face environment.

This doesn't mean that online learning is more effective than classroom learning, but it does suggest that there are certain advantages in online learning.

A student studying online under an expert tutor may do better than one who studies in a class taught by an average or below average tutor.

This observation is significantly supported if the online learning is performed for a continuous term, in compared with a sporadic term spent weekly in a class environment. In addition, online tutor is always available, whereas the classroom teacher is not.

Evidence for the benefits of online learning does not make classroom teaching obsolete, but it will prompt the introduction of more techniques and tools for online learning and extend the areas in which it is used.

A clear benefit of making extensive use of online learning would be the significant reduction of the cost of learning that would result.

Online educational and technological developments will also have a significant impact on students and teachers.

In the future teachers will have better online tools and will require specialised training to be able to use them effectively.

Another relatively new trend in education is home-schooling. Home-schooling is growing throughout the world, but particularly in the USA.

Families who home-school their children are independent of public funding and take responsibility for the full cost of their children's education. This means that home-schooling represents a significant saving to the taxpayer. The triangular relationship linking teacher, parent and student should be strengthened through cooperation, monitoring and feedback.

It is vital to emphasise that all parties have share a common goal and that close cooperation can help to achieve that goal. Some parents take a hands-off approach to their child's education or decide not to get involved in school events as their children grow up.

The evidence which has accumulated suggests that this is generally not a desirable approach; it is recommended that parents take an active role their children's education. Attentive parents will quickly notice any changes in their children's demeanour or behaviour, but teachers should also report any changes in a student's behaviour or any other changes which make affect his or her education to parents. There is no question that children's performance improves when they know that their parents are involved and support their school activities.

Conversely if a child feels that his or her parents and teacher are not united in their attitudes and opinions it may have a detrimental effect on his or her behaviour and academic achievement.

Both parents and teachers can see the global picture, at home and in school, but the student will be concerned with small details of his or her early life in a relatively new social environment.

The need to make new friends and sometimes also to leave old friends can have a significant psychological impact on a child. Adapting to a new school environment can be difficult, especially when the class is large and some of ones classmates are rather hostile.

More attention should be given to developmental differences between boys and girls. Neuroscientists have uncovered evidence of differences between the brains of boys and girls and linked these to their academic abilities and learning preferences.

As a result some people recommend single-sex education, at least until the eighth grade; however this is not a strategy endorsed by the majority of educators. Parents should make an effort to reduce noise and other problems that may impede our child's learning.

It is therefore is essential that the triangle of parents, teacher and student is a stable one.

Educational inequalities are becoming more extreme, i.e. the gap between the educated and the non-educated is increasing over time.

New educational systems may be developed around realistic scenarios and events and not necessarily based only on its basic components. This may lead to an interdisciplinary education enabling the analysis and the comprehension of real-life events.

In other words, in order to improve understanding of real-world events and equip students to apply their knowledge in real-world context one might develop a more applied, interdisciplinary approach to education, making greater use of realistic scenarios and placing more emphasis on applied rather than abstract knowledge.

In a homogeneous society without private education options access to education is more equal.

The fact that the social upper class has access to special educational tools such as private lessons may increase the social inequality in education.

We should use multidisciplinary art, antiques and collectables as intellectual stimulation.

Combining several such multidisciplinary elements with psychological tools might help to reduce crime. We all are aware that crime reduction is one of the main goals of public policy.

It is obvious that a reduction in crime would have economic and social benefits. In a difficult financial environment shifting resources from crime fighting to education can be recommended as it may be a more effective crime fighting strategy.

Some claim that school is a microcosm of society and that more education doesn't necessarily produce more law-abiding citizens. There is some truth in that claim, but the question is, can we do anything about it?

In other words, can we do anything about the fact that more education doesn't necessarily produce more law-abiding citizens?

I believe that we can.

In problem communities investing in and supervising early childhood education may lead to a reduction in crime in that community later on.

A crime reduction strategy requires that we introduce another element into the parent-teacher-student triangle, namely the police supported by the government, who are responsible for policy making.

Crime research should not focus solely on individual students but also on problematic teachers.

Teachers, who should be authority figures, sometimes abuse their power and discriminate in a way which may affect students' reactions to an event.

Teachers have a responsibility to generate a good learning atmosphere and create bonds between students as well as just instructing them.

This should be done without any prejudice and in a way which is independent of social class, academic ability or ethnicity.

In order to create positive and supportive society we have to nurture our children and encourage them to feel positive about themselves and their peers in school. School teachers should encourage students to volunteer for civic duties and promote an appreciation for the law and its implications.

This kind of environment would not only have a beneficial effect on learning but it might also lead to a reduction in crime down the line. Academic success or failure is not solely in the hands of the student.

Parents have a responsibility to provide a suitable environment for learning and teachers should identify any problems the student has and try to resolve them. In certain socialist countries, particularly before the 1980s, a student's failure was considered to be the teacher's failure. The teacher would be obliged to stay after school hours, without extra pay, to go over material with students who had had difficulty absorbing and understanding it in class. There was a universal intolerance of failure in school.

20. FUTURE TEACHING METHODS.

FROM TIME TO TIME we hear about novel teaching methods, which may be effective in certain circumstances or for a specific age group or subject.

Developing techniques or tools which make learning interesting and stimulating and may increase children's motivation to learn is an important and commendable task.

In preschool education games can be a very useful aid to teaching. If they are well-designed children may learn without even realising that they are doing so.

Teacher should take advantage of students' engagement with social media to introduce new knowledge and skills via social networking systems.

We should also encourage small-group learning method; using brainstorming and analysing scenarios to develop new and original ideas.

Obviously, one of the important forms of learning is autodidacticism or self-learning.

The major stimulating factor to succeed in self-learning is by nurturing and enhancing student's curiosity. In other words, the most important determinant of autodidactic learning is curiosity, and so to promote autodidacticism we should nurture students' sense of curiosity.

Over time the amount of information available in the world is increasing; the burden this imposes on students is obvious.

With the explosion in information it will become more and more difficult to learn everything and sometimes it will be sufficient to know of the existence and location of a piece of information.

My prediction is that brain implants will become available, and, in combination with online learning will make face-to-face teaching redundant.

We will need new education laws to accommodate this kind of technological progress.

If and when we work out how our brain stores information there will be a global educational revolution. I envisage the development of sophisticated new 'edu-capsules' each type dedicated to a particular subject. Such a biotechnological breakthrough has the potential to make our entire educational system redundant and could have a devastating impact on governments across the world.

Any such revolutionary change in education should therefore be implemented gradually and with great care; we must learn from historical revolutions.

The introduction of machines and automation led to the significant changes in the labour force. There were large-scale redundancies and workers had to be re-educated to carry out different and more skilled tasks. Something similar may happen in educational systems.

The history of education shows that teachers throughout the world have had to cope with significant changes.

Changes in demography, technology, religion and other factors have required teachers to adapt and update their skills and practices to cope. Special attention should be paid to educators, their position in the society and their ability to educate and as well as simply passing on information.

If we reach the stage where knowledge can simply be implanted in the brain our social life will also be revolutionised, just as it was by the introduction of Facebook in 2000.

We may find ourselves asking if we still need schools and teachers.

I believe that we will need a completely different type of educational system that can accommodate and manage technological developments for the benefit of a new interdisciplinary society.

21. BOOKS BY DR. GIORA RAM (English):

Nuke Them Till Eternity (prev. The Hungarian Connection)
An Autobiographical Novel.
Published in Israel by IMEXCO General Ltd, 2010, 2018
ISBN 978-965-91623-9-0 | Paperback and Kindle formats on Amazon
http://nuke.imexco.com

Sex and Scientific Philosophy
A unique collection of earthly and heavenly questions arising during
our intellectual evolution.
Published in Israel by IMEXCO General Ltd, 2012
ISBN 978-965-91623-1-4 | Paperback and Kindle formats on Amazon
http://philosex.imexco.com

**Hunting for Antiques and Collectables: The Adventures of an
Antique Collector**
Hunting adventures for unique and rare antiques and collectables
Published in Israel by IMEXCO General Ltd, 2013
ISBN 978-965-91623-2-1 | Paperback and Kindle formats on Amazon
http://aoc.imexco.com ; http://antiques.imexco.com

Evolutionary and Philosophical Insights into Global Education
This book is in two parts. In part one, the focus is on past and
present educational methods and systems whilst part two contains
forward-looking views and opinions on educational needs and
possible new forms of information transfer.
Published in Israel by IMEXCO General Ltd, 2015
ISBN 978-965-91623-3-8 | Paperback and Kindle formats on Amazon
http://edu.imexco.com

Education and Alternative Treatments for ADHD
A unique methodological non-drug-based treatment successfully
implemented on the author's son is presented here in conjunction
with global education related issues.
Published in Israel by IMEXCO General Ltd, 2015, 2018
ISBN 978-965-91623-6-9 | Paperback and Kindle formats on Amazon
http://adhd.imexco.com

Articles in English
https://ezinearticles.com/expert/Dr_Giora_Ram/1368314

Books by Dr. Giora Ram (Hebrew):

ADHD - Children of Tomorrow
A unique co-production of a special child and his father.
Published in Israel by Gvanim, 2010
DanaCode 00860000644-6 | Paperback and Kindle formats on Amazon
http://adhd.imexco.com

The House on the Hill
Poems and Love Letters
Published in Israel by IMEXCO General Ltd, 2010
DanaCode 08000250081-4 | Paperback and Kindle formats on Amazon
http://love-u.imexco.com

My Love, My Wife, My Divorcee
Dating and mating
Published in Israel by IMEXCO General Ltd, 2010
DanaCode 08000250082-1 | Paperback and Kindle formats on Amazon
http://my-love.imexco.com

Mr. Giggle the Story Teller
Adventures in the world of dreams
Published in Israel by IMEXCO General Ltd, 2016
ISBN 978-965-91623-5-2 | Paperback and Kindle formats on Amazon
http://mrgiggle.imexco.com

A Tale of Love and Passion for Life
What would a retired Mossad agent do when he discovers that he
has a terminal cancer and has only three more months left to live?
This novel is based on the turbulent exciting life of a Mossad agent.
Published in Israel by IMEXCO General Ltd, 2016
ISBN 978-965-91623-4-5 | Paperback format on Amazon
http://passion4life.imexco.com

Stories and Poems about Love and Life
This book contains a collection of short stories written by the author
during the last decade. They were published in various media.
Published in Israel by Dr. Giora Ram, 2017
ISBN 978-965-91623-7-6 | Paperback format on Amazon
http://stories.imexco.com

Articles in Hebrew: https://www.articles.co.il/authorFB/28455